Is It A Cold Or The Flu?

How to Recognize the Difference and Treat the Flu Naturally

RON KNESS

Published by:

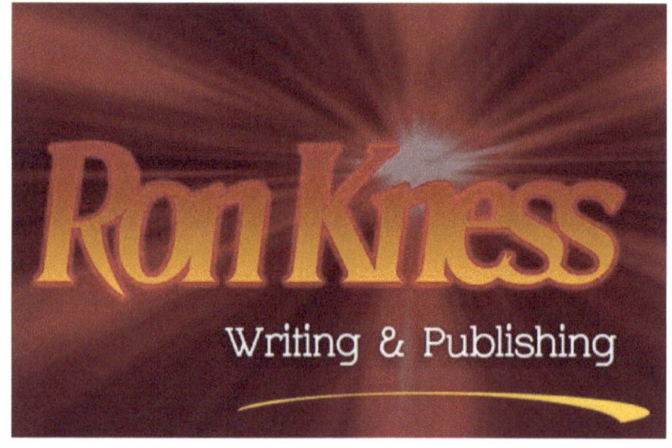

Gold Canyon, AZ

United States of America

ISBN-13: 978-1983656002

ISBN-10: 1983656003

Contents

Disclaimer

This publication is for informational purposes only and is not intended as medical advice. Medical advice should always be obtained from a qualified medical professional for any health conditions or symptoms associated with them.

Every possible effort has been made in preparing and researching this material. We make no warranties with respect to the accuracy, applicability of its contents or any omissions.

See your healthcare professional before starting any diet, health or exercise program!

Introduction

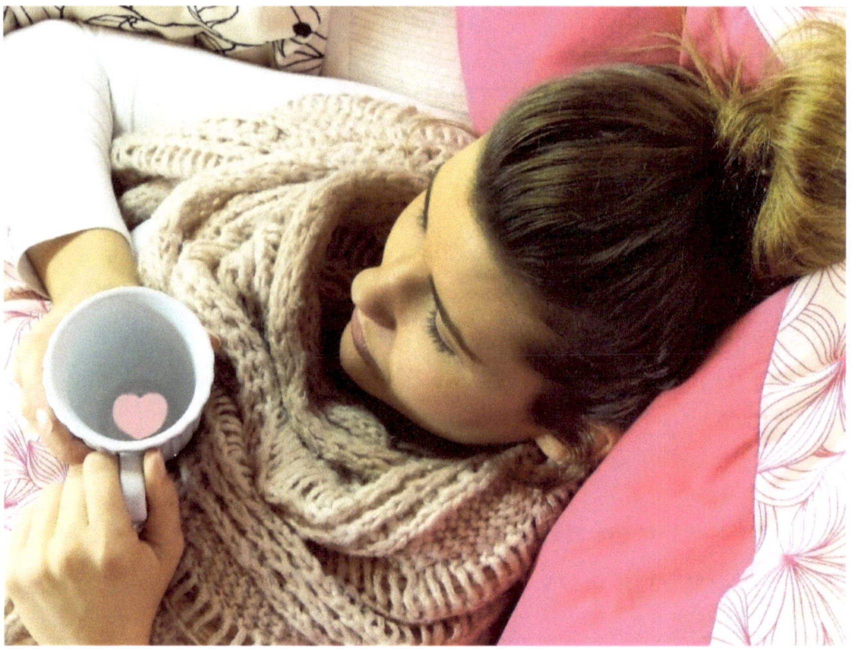

What are the differences between a cold and the flu? One of the most confusing things about becoming sick with an upper respiratory illness such as a cold or the flu is that they begin in a similar manner. However, each requires a different treatment to limit the illness and get over it as quickly as possible.

A Cold

A cold is caused by becoming infected with a rhinovirus. Like many viruses, it mutates. There are hundreds of strains of the common cold virus and any of them can be around at any time. New strains can form all the time, making it difficult to build up immunity to them.

Viruses have no cure, but you can treat the symptoms as best you can to make you or your loved ones more comfortable if they come down with a cold.

Typical symptoms of a cold include:

- Congestion (head and/or chest)

- Runny nose (stuffiness from swollen sinuses)

- Watery eyes

- Coughing - it can be a dry cough, or one that is productive, that is, produces phlegm in order to get congestion out of your body

- Headache

- Tiredness

- Itchy nose, eyes and throat

- Fever (more common in children)

- Sore throat

The Flu

The flu is caused by becoming infected with one of the strains of the influenza virus.

The flu generally comes on more quickly than a cold. The symptoms seem to hit all at once, and will usually be more severe than when you catch a cold.

The typical symptoms of flu include:

- Runny or stuffy nose

- Cough

- Sore throat

- Headaches and/or body aches

- Fever or feeling feverish (not everyone with the flu has a fever)

- Chills

- Fatigue, lack of energy

- Nausea, vomiting

- Diarrhea (most common in children)

While the first four symptoms are common to both flu and colds, they are likely to be more intense when you have the flu. Flu symptoms are strong right from the onset, and they usually run their course in about a week. Colds usually only last a few days.

Flu Symptoms and How it Spreads

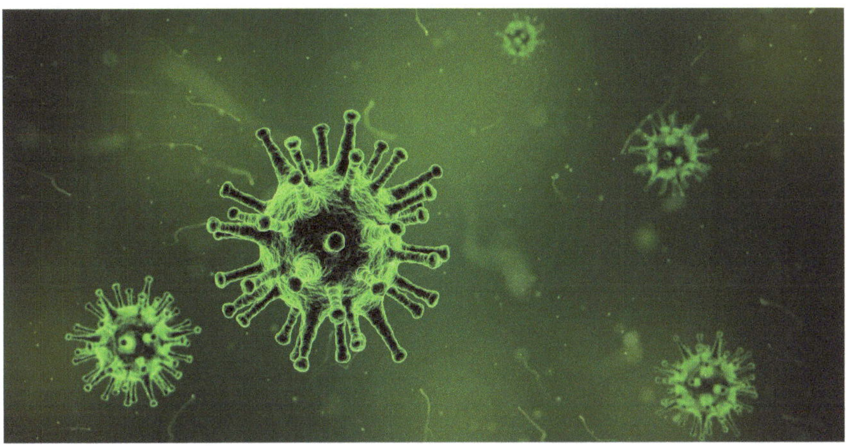

Influenza symptoms include fever, cough, headaches, chills, body aches, a sore throat and fatigue. Vomiting and diarrhea are usually not reported with a respiratory-type of flu. However, the drainage from the sinus cavities and mucus production can cause an upset tummy. The illness lasts from one to two weeks depending on the health of the individual and if treatment is started with antiviral medications.

It is important to remember that the common cold has many of the same symptoms. However, the onset of the flu is usually much more severe and quicker than with the common cold. You go to bed with mild symptoms in the evening and wake up with the full blown flu the next morning. Cold symptoms last about 7 days with a gradual onset and the decrease of symptoms.

It is important to remember that flu is not a rare illness. According to estimates from the Centers for Disease Control, www.cdc.gov, 5 to 20 percent of the U.S. population suffers from a case of the flu each year.

Flu is similar to a cold virus in that it is typically spread from one person to another when an infected person coughs or sneezes. The virus can pass out through an infected person's lungs, throat or nose, sending particles into the air that can pass to anyone that person comes in close contact with. The range to pass the infection is from 3 to 6 feet.

Being out in a crowd increases your chances of being infected, because the more people you're exposed to, the higher the probability that several of them have the beginning stages of the flu. Additionally the closer people are next to each other, the less distance the virus has to travel when airborne.

Being in an airplane in the closed environment with someone who has the flu makes it more likely the flu spreads to the other passengers. Transportation by bus or subway increases the close approximation between passengers.

The other main way the virus spreads is from touching surfaces that are contaminated with the virus and then touching your eyes, mouth or nose. An individual infected with the virus can start transmitting it up to a day before the symptoms start, and up to a week after the symptoms become noticeable, according to the Centers for Disease Control. The flu virus remains active for up to 24 hours on hard surfaces and about 12 hours on soft surfaces. You may pick up the flu virus if you touch the contaminated surface and then touch your face.

Preventing the Spread of the Flu

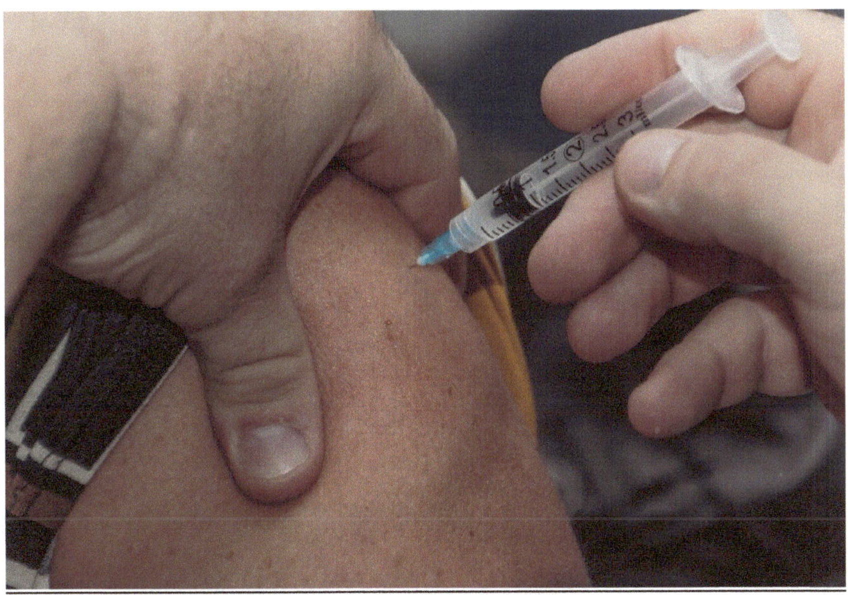

For the sake of our own health and others, we all have a responsibility to prevent the spread of flu, or any other type of disease for that matter. It doesn't take a rocket scientist or brain surgeon to figure out what to do; most of the steps are common sense.

As noted before, from 5 to 20% of the population in the US comes down with the flu every year. While most of us get through the flu just fine, it can be a serious disease for the young and old.

Cover your nose or mouth when you sneeze or cough, so you trap the virus particles in the tissue rather than expelling them into the air. Then make sure you dispose of the tissue so it won't spread the virus on any other surface. The flu virus is spread within a 3 to 6 foot diameter when you sneeze so trapping the virus in a tissue eliminates that possibility.

After you sneeze or cough, wash your hands with soap and water. Or if you are not near a sink, use an alcohol-based hand cleaner. Get in the habit of carrying these hand sanitizers with you, in the car, in your pocket or in your purse. Ensure the one you use has at least 62% alcohol. Wash or disinfect your hands when out in the public and touching door knobs, shopping cart handles or other items that other people touch.

Avoid touching your mouth, nose or eyes. If you have touched any object contaminated with the virus, you may end up contaminating yourself. Your eyes, nose and mouth are the easiest pathways to infection by the flu virus.

If you're sick, stay home from work and away from other people. You may think that you're being Mr. Tough Guy by going into work, but you won't be working at full capacity when you're sick and you'll be spreading the flu virus. If your child becomes sick, keep them home from school until their symptoms have subsided. You can spread the flu from a day or so before you exhibit symptoms until you're well. Most flu symptoms last from one to two weeks.

The medical community encourages everyone to get a flu vaccine every year. The virus mutates a bit from year to year, so last year's immunization may not protect you from this year's virus. And the vaccine isn't always effective.

About 40 to 60% of the population that get vaccinated still get the flu. However, it's usually is a milder case and doesn't last as long.

Handwashing Number 1 in Preventing the Flu

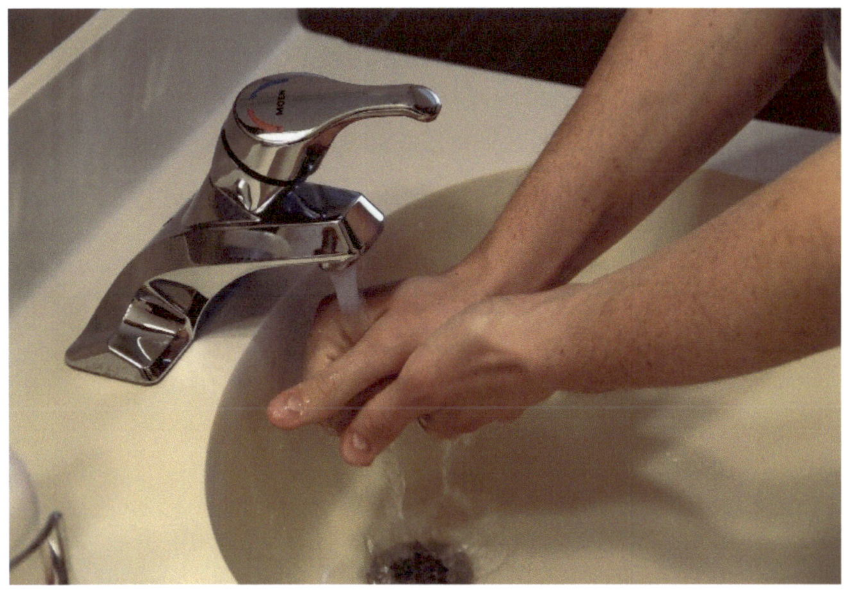

No one likes to be sick with the flu but it happens. While you'd have to lock yourself in an air bubble away from other people to guarantee that you won't get sick from the flu, there are ways to decrease your chances of becoming infected. Frequent hand washing is one of the easiest and best measures you can take to reduce your chance of coming down with the flu.

During the day all of us touch dozens of surfaces that may have the flu virus on them: doorknobs, grocery cart handles, computer mouse and keyboards, cell phones and telephones—the list is endless. The virus remains active on hard surfaces for up to 24 hours. And don't think that if no one in your family is exhibiting flu symptoms, you're in the clear.

You can be contagious for a couple of days before you become sick.

Wash your hands with hot soapy water, dry with a paper towel and throw the towel away. When in public restrooms, be careful of the surfaces you touch. If the restroom has a hot air hand dryer, use that instead of paper towels. Antibacterial soap isn't necessary as the flu is caused by a virus not bacteria. It won't be killed by the soap. It will be destroyed by the hot water and the friction from rubbing your hands together with the soap.

If soap and water isn't available, use an alcohol based hand sanitizer instead. Again rubbing causes friction and that friction kills the virus. Don't dry the hand sanitizer off with a paper towel. Let your hands dry naturally. That gives the alcohol more time to work.

It is important to instruct children in these preventive measures as well. Children come in contact with more potential sources of germs, including flu viruses, than adults do. Not only do they have a classroom of up to 40 other children, but they make contact with other children outside their class at lunch time and on the playground.

The immune systems of children aren't as developed as adults so they get sick more often. Teaching your child to wash their hands often is one of the best ways to prevent them from becoming ill. Give each child their own bottle of hand sanitizer to carry with them, if it's allowed by the school rules.

If you conscientiously wash your hands after touching potentially contaminated surfaces you and your family may be able to squeak through this flu season without becoming ill.

After You Come Down With the Flu

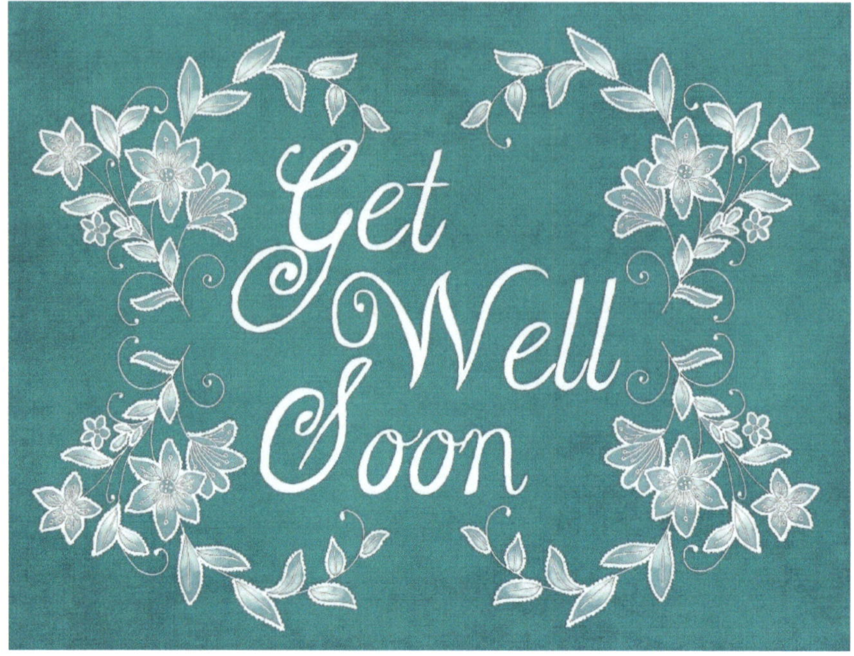

Flu season is here with the coughing, headache, congestion, sore throat and runny nose. It's a miserable time to get sick especially with the cold, wet windy weather outside. Let's face it: winter and early spring are the flu season with it peaking in most places around February.

Having the flu is one instance where you must stay home from work, school or other social situations where you could spread the virus. Your recovery from the illness will be accelerated if you allow yourself plenty of rest, rather than trying to keep with your normal work schedule. If you must work while you are recovering, do it via computer or telephone from home and limit it to a few hours each day.

Do not travel on public transportation when you are sick. The confined space of an airplane, or bus, for example, makes it quite possible that whenever you sneeze or cough, and you will, other passengers become infected. Since the flu virus is airborne for up to 6 feet, which means in a crowded bus you could infect four or five other people with every sneeze.

Stay prepared during the flu season. Make sure you have lots of fruit juice, light meals, and tissues on hand. Being sick and having to go to the store makes you feel worse and exposes others to your illness.

Pack up an emergency flu kit in an empty shoe box so you know where everything is. You'll need aspirin, saline nasal spray, tissues, plastic sealable baggies to put the used tissues in, hand sanitizer, throat lozenges, bottled water, tea bags and the citrus juices. Sports drinks work but keep in mind that they can contain sugar, salt and caffeine. If you like also include a decongestant, and cough medicine.

You might also want to have instant soups on hand. The warmth and salt in the soups will sooth your throat and help clear congestion.

A humidifier is helpful as well. During winter when home heating systems are going full blast the air is dry and can irritate nasal passages. A humidifier in the room adds much needed moisture so you can breathe easier.

Remember that this too shall pass. Flu symptoms are worse in the first few days of the illness and become milder later in the week. Most flu symptoms are gone within a week to 10 days. Take your time and don't rush yourself trying to get better. The odds are you'll suffer a relapse.

What to Do If A Family Member Comes Down With the Flu

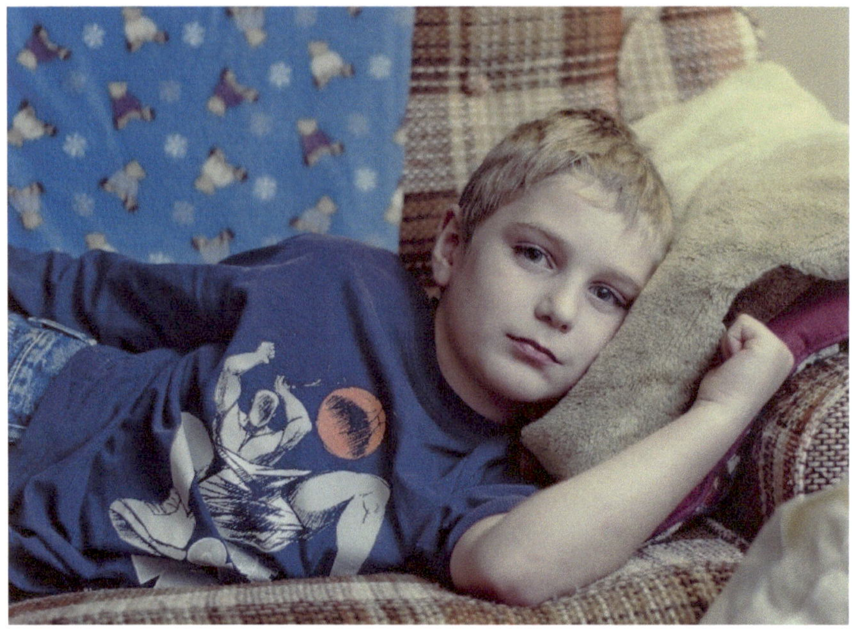

If a family member comes down with the flu, take steps to make sure it doesn't spread throughout the household. Just because one member is sick doesn't mean the whole family has to get sick. Frequently disinfect the bathroom surfaces, doorknobs or other areas the family member suffering from the flu may have touched. Keep their toothbrush separate from other family members'. Make sure family members don't accidentally share drinking glasses.

Keep the patient home. Going to work or school just spreads the flu to more victims. The odds are the patient isn't going to be very productive even if they choose to go to work, so why not stay home and work on getting well instead.

Call the school to see if any work can be brought home for the patient when they feel a little better.

Working at home is an option for those who can telecommute. Just remember that lots of rest is important to getting better.

Any area the infected person may have touched or coughed or sneezed on must be disinfected as long as the person is contagious, which can be as long as two weeks. Even something as routine as family members drying their hands with the same towel can be a means of spreading the virus. Use paper towels in the bathroom and kitchen. Keeping your home as germ and virus free as possible year round is one of the best ways to make sure the possibility of family members becoming infected is minimized.

Keep a container of disinfectant wipes prominently displayed on the bathroom and kitchen counters. Instruct everyone to wipe down the door handles, faucet handles and counter tops whenever they use the bathroom. Sprays are messier and have to be wiped off anyway so the disinfectant wipes are better.

Buy bottles of hand sanitizer and place one in every room. There no excuse for not using it when it's right there. Do the same thing with a box of tissues. Sneezing is a main culprit in the spread of the flu virus.

Keep a thermos filled with hot tea or other warm liquids, along with a carafe of water and perhaps a couple of bottles of juice by the patient. Keeping hydrated is important. If the liquid is right by the bedside, your patient may be more likely to keep drinking.

Keep an eye on the patient for worsening symptoms. While most of us get over the flu without any complications, others don't. Symptoms should start getting less intense after the first few days. If they worsen, it could be a sign of secondary infections. The very young and seniors are more prone to complications. Influenza kills 36,000 people in the US every year according to the Center for Disease Control.

Flu Prevention: Does Vitamin C Prevent the Flu?

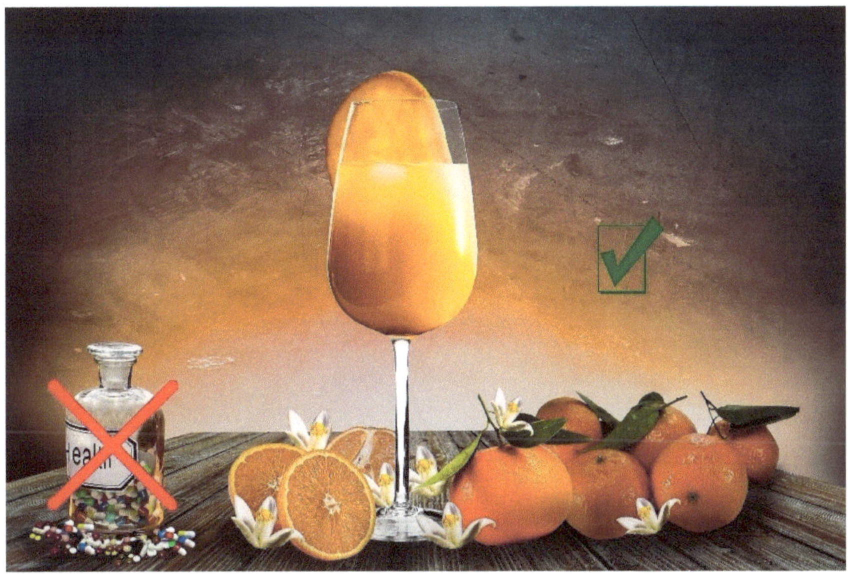

It's cold and windy, you have the sniffles and think you might be coming down with a cold or even worse, the flu. If you're worried about contracting the flu should you take extra Vitamin C?

There are not any studies that have shown the Vitamin C prevents the flu or any other flu virus, shortens its duration or makes the illness milder. However, what Vitamin C does do is strengthen the immune system. Since the immune system is how the body fights off any virus, maintaining a strong immune system makes sense. Vitamin C boosts the production of white blood cells, antibodies and interferon, all of which are critical to fighting the flu and lots of other illnesses.

Keep in mind that most drug studies are conducted by pharmaceutical companies with the idea that if the drug is successful, the drug company can patent the drug and make a nice profit. Vitamin C can't be patented, so there isn't much of an incentive for the studies about its effectiveness to be completed.

Vitamin C is found naturally in many foods such as oranges, lemons, limes, strawberries, and leafy greens. One of the best sources of Vitamin C is kiwi fruit. One small kiwi fruit has twice the Vitamin C as a medium orange. Many foods are fortified with Vitamin C, and of course it's available as a supplement.

Since the vitamin is water soluble it is not stored in the body. Any excess over what the body requires for that day is excreted out in the urine. However more isn't always better; any substance can be toxic if too much is taken at any one time, even water. For example: drinking extreme amounts of water can throw off the electrolyte balance of the body.

How much vitamin C is recommended? Sixty mg is the recommended daily amount. However the body's requirement varies depending on age, activity level, and exposure. For example, people under stress, and smokers, require more. Many people believe that 500 mg is the optimum dosage. An orange has 70 mg of vitamin C. It would be a challenge to consume 500 mg just through foods. To get that amount from just oranges alone, you would have to eat at least seven oranges.

While vitamin C hasn't been shown to prevent the flu, it's still a good idea to make sure you and your family get enough through diet and supplements during the flu season.

It makes sense to increase your level a few weeks before flu season and continue for a few weeks after flu season. That's approximately the winter months with a couple of weeks on either side.

Is the Flu Virus Killed by Ultraviolet light?

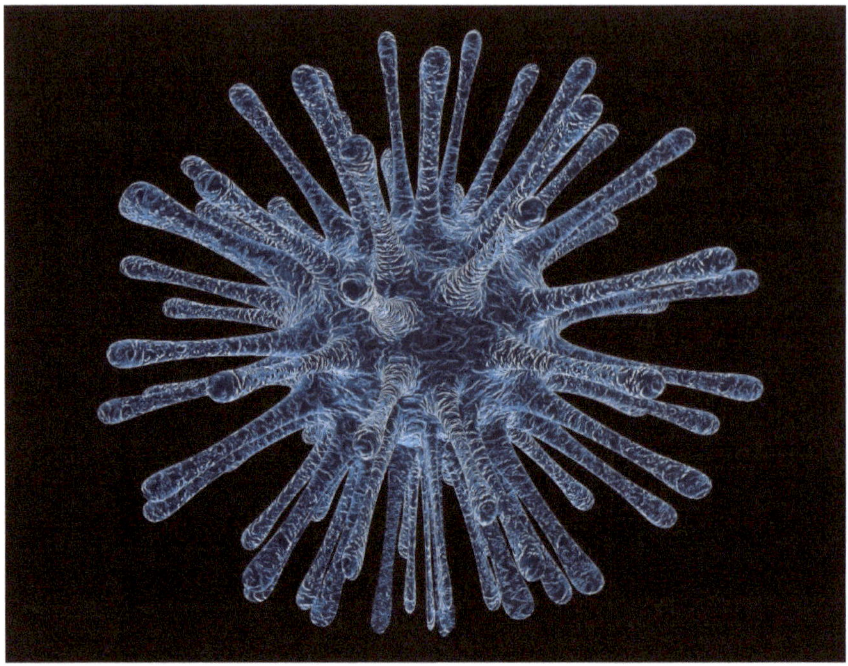

The flu season is here and lasts from winter on through early spring. Seasonal flu viruses are more of a threat to those under 5 years old or over 60 years or those who already have health problems, but they cause everyone discomfort and time lost from school or work. If you're worried about contracting the flu, are there more precautions you can take besides washing your hands or using a hand sanitizing gel?

Viruses are not alive the way a plant or an animal is alive. They do not consume, excrete waste product, grow, or react to their environment. They do however reproduce themselves, but only in a host cell.

The virus is dormant outside the host cell and can live on inanimate articles up to 24 hours.

A specific type of virus will only reproduce in a specific type of host cell. In other words if you're a rose plant, you can't get tobacco mosaic virus. There are viruses that affect just about every type of organism.

Viruses are the cause of the flu, ebola, HIV, rabies, herpes, the common cold, measles, chicken pox, polio, and more. Viruses are dangerous because they mutate; the mutation means that previous vaccines are useless against the new strain. It also means the new strain can be far more devastating in the damage it cause. The flu of 1917 started out as a flu with mild symptoms, mutated, and killed nearly 50 million people worldwide in a relatively short period of time.

Ultraviolet light used in water purifiers and air filters does deactivate or kill viruses. Ultraviolet light represents the frequency of light between 200 nanometers (nm) and 400 nm. You can't see it with the naked eye. The most effective frequency for killing viruses and bacteria is at the lower end of the scale - between 254 nm and 265 nm.

The viruses are deactivated because the light causes genetic damage. The virus can no longer reproduce itself. Ultraviolet lights used in home filters need to be wiped off every six months. Some systems are closed and signal that the bulb needs to be changed. They use about the same amount of energy as a 40-watt incandescent bulb.

Should you use an air filter that uses ultraviolet light? That depends on how often you're exposed to people who may be sick, how much the air in your home is circulated, and other factors.   Many modern homes are virtually sealed air systems in the winter when the heat is on or during the summer with air conditioning. This closed system doesn't allow the viruses to dissipate but keeps them trapped within your home.

Decrease Stress and Decrease the Odds of Getting the Flu

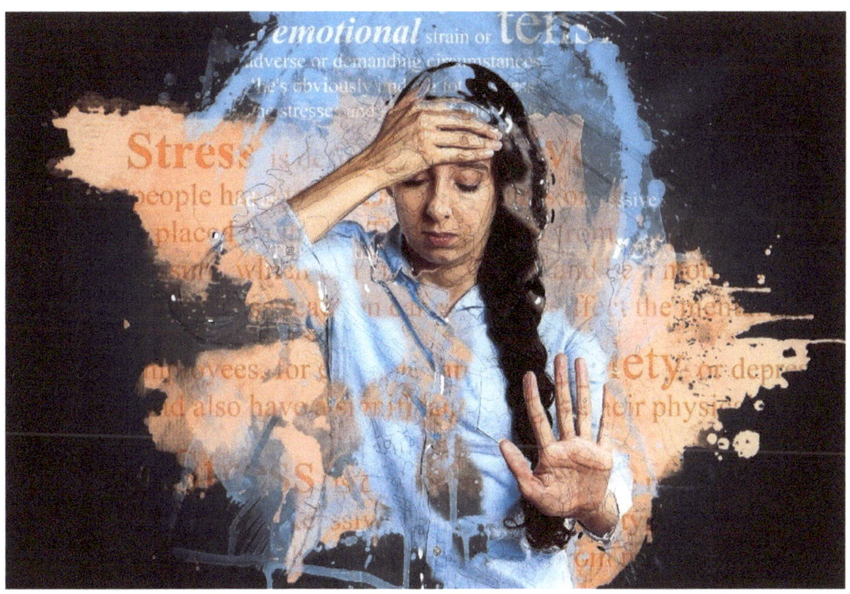

Stress in modern day life is nearly impossible to avoid even without the worries of whether you'll come down with the flu. Stress makes the body more susceptible to becoming infected with a virus. The immune system has to deal with the stress as well as attempt to keep invaders like the influenza virus from infecting the body. Here are a few tips to decrease stress in your life:

<u>Take a few minutes for quiet time</u>

We're surrounded by noise. The TV's always going. The radio gets turned on the moment we get in the car. The loud speakers blare as we grocery shop. It's a noisy world and that noise can add to stress levels. Enjoy the peacefulness of quiet. Intentionally spend 15 to 30 minutes in peaceful silence.

You don't even have to do anything but listen to the silence if you don't want to.

Start Your Day on a Positive Note

Don't get bogged down by last night's dishes, early morning laundry chores or racing around the house to get yourself ready for work. That's just starting your day loaded with stress. Start the day by reading a few pages from your favorite inspirational book. Have a cup of coffee (https://www.amazon.com/Discover-Health-Benefits-Coffee-Science/dp/1547188979) on your back porch looking at the sun rise. Take a few moments and write in your journal (https://journalingforfun.com). The world will wait and you will be ready for it.

Take Time for Yourself Every Day

Do something you enjoy every day. It can be something as simple as taking a walk with your puppy pal, or stroking your kitty cat. Value yourself by giving yourself a treat. If you love to garden but just haven't had the time, make the time. Buy an assortment of herbs and pots and potter for a bit. Doing something you like is a great stress buster.

Practice Meditation

You don't have to sit there in the lotus position and hum for 30 minutes to meditate. Choose a place that is quiet and pleasant. It can be in your garden, your favorite chair or even on the floor in your bedroom. Close your eyes and focus on a pleasant feeling. For example, if you love going to the beach and watching the waves roll onto the shore, focus on that feeling.

After even five minutes you'll feel more relaxed. You can't prevent the flu, but you can decrease the odds that you'll get it if you de-stress your life.

3 Ways to Cut Down the Chances of Getting the Flu

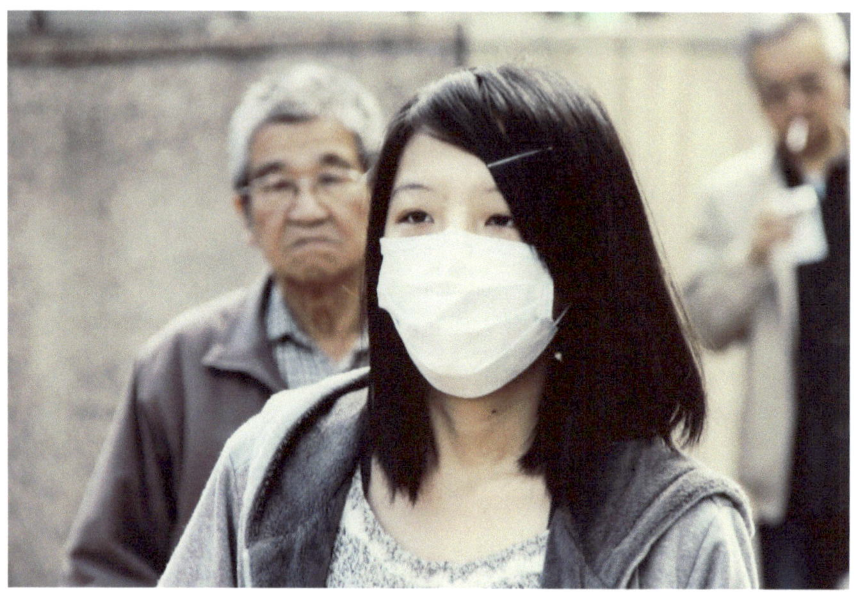

Winter time is flu season. There's just no way around it. But just because the flu is going around doesn't mean you have to become infected. While the only way to completely prevent the flu is to isolate yourself from friends, family and the public, you can cut down on the chances of you becoming sick. There are several common sense ways you can get down the chances of coming down with flu.

1. **Wash your hands**. A lot. It's one of the best and most effective ways to prevent disease. Wash your hands for at least 20 seconds using warm to hot water and soap. It doesn't have to be an antibacterial soap because the flu is caused by a virus not a bacteria. The virus won't be killed. The heat from the water and rubbing your hands together gets rid of the virus.

If you're out and about and don't have access to soap and water, use a hand sanitizer gel that is alcohol based. Use a generous dollop and rub on your hands until it evaporates. Wash your hands after you've been out in public.

2. **Stay away from crowds**. The flu is airborne within a 6 foot distance. The virus is carried on water droplets that are expelled from the nasal passages, throat and lungs through sneezing, coughing and breathing. If you aren't where the crowds are - you won't be exposed as much.

If the flu season is especially bad and you're in the more at risk groups because of your age or damaged immune system, consider wearing an air filter mask when you're in crowds. Make sure you wash your hands after you remove the mask.

3. **Don't touch your mouth or nose with your hands, use a tissue.** The flu is spread through the virus being introduced to the host - that's you. If the virus is on your hand because you touched a surface that someone else did who had the virus and then touch your nose or mouth, you increase the chances of getting sick yourself. Use the tissue only once and throw it away after usage.

Don't touch door handles in public areas if you can help it, or stair rails, even grocery shopping carts can carry the virus for a while. Many grocery stores now provide disinfectant wipes to clean the handles of the cart. Use these common sense rules to decrease the chance you'll get sick from flu.

Keep The Flu Virus at Bay With a Healthy Lifestyle

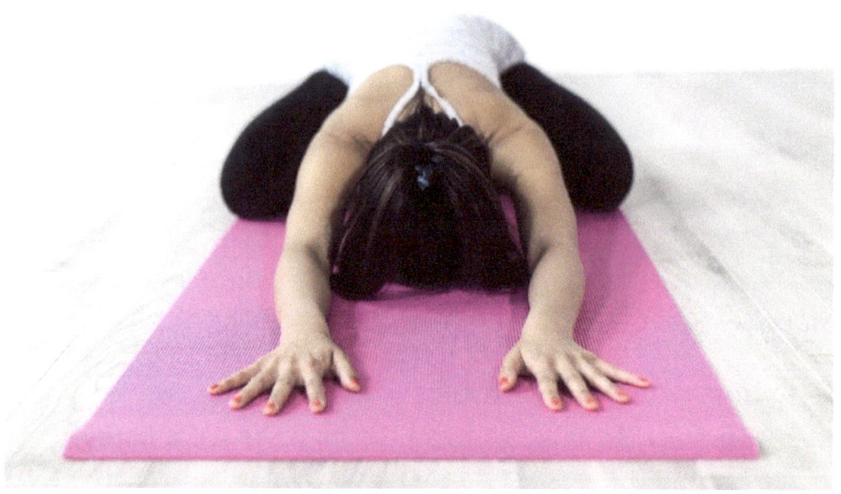

One of the reasons the human body is so amazing is that it is always dealing with threats, such as infection from bacteria or viruses—but most of the time we don't get sick because our immune system is working 24/7 to combat these threats.

Having a healthy immune system (https://www.amazon.com/Power-Your-Immune-System-Year-round/dp/1534842349) is one of the reasons many of us don't succumb to illness even during the normal cold and flu seasons of the year. Conversely, bad lifestyle habits can seriously weaken our immune systems and make us more susceptible to infection.

It is generally accepted that a number of factors completely under our control can help boost our immune systems. Eating a balanced diet is one element of keeping your immune system strong.

This includes making sure you get the right balance and dosage of vitamins, either from our diet or from vitamin supplements.

We are often told that when we're sick we should drink plenty of fluids, but drinking sufficient fluids is actually something we should do every day to help us prevent getting sick in the first place. Liquids help the body flush toxins from the system.

Many times, germs such as the flu are swept from our respiratory system before they have a chance to multiply and cause us to become ill. All liquids count but water is the cheapest and most convenient.

Getting plenty of sleep is important. Fatigue makes it more difficult for your body to repair itself. Regular exercise is important not just for disease prevention in the short run but to make sure we maintain good health throughout our lives. Chronic high levels of stress is thought to contribute to weakening the immune system, so employing stress management techniques not only can help us feel better mentally, but may also help our immune system work at top efficiency.

The flu is caused by a virus, so don't think that taking a course of antibiotics will lessen the symptoms or prevent infection. It won't. Antibiotics have no effect on the flu virus or any virus for that matter. Antibiotics are effective in killing bacteria.

What may be a little confusing is that your body produces antibodies against the virus when infected. But antibodies are not at all the same thing as antibiotics. A strong healthy body produces lots of antibodies when invaded by the flu.

A positive lifestyle (https://www.amazon.com/Healthy-Lifestyle-Diet-Eating-Longevity/dp/1543240585) can boost the odds of staying healthy and avoiding not only the flu but other types of diseases.

Avoiding--and Dealing With--Flu in the Workplace

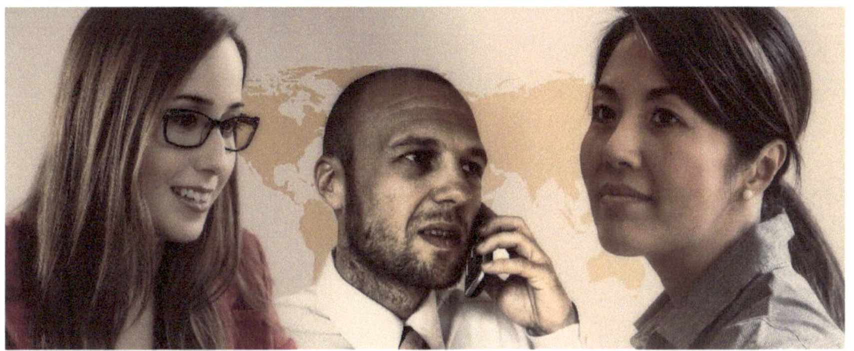

Because in most workplaces you are in close proximity with other people, some of who may be already sick or coming down with the flu, it is easy to pick up the flu virus while at work. While you can't eliminate your chances of getting the flue while at work, here are five things you can do to lessen your chances.

Get Plenty of Rest

This is good advice year-round to maintain good health and be as productive as possible in your career. But during flu season, rest is especially important to keep your immune system strong and lower the chances of being infected. Don't over-work yourself to the point of fatigue. Putting in long hours won't do you any good if it results in your losing a week of work because you get sick.

Wash and Sanitize Hands and Surfaces

We all touch many surfaces each day, from door knobs to keyboards, and have no way of knowing which of these might have flu virus on them. Wash your hands with warm soapy water whenever you come into contact with objects or surfaces that co-workers have touched. If soap isn't available, use hand sanitizer.

Make a habit of carrying a small bottle of sanitizer with you and keeping one in your desk. Anti-bacterial soap is not effective at killing viruses. The key to hand washing is to rub your hands vigorously, which destroys the viruses. Desks, door knobs and other surfaces should be rubbed with sanitizing wipes designed to kill viruses.

Encourage Those Infected with Flu to Stay Home from Work--Including Yourself

Think about how many people you come in contact with during a typical work day. If you are in the stage where you can transmit the flu virus to others, you can spread the virus through airborne contamination every time you sneeze or cough. No one would want to spread the flu misery to co-workers. That's why being at work when you are sick is not heroic, it's foolish.

If you see an employee or co-worker suffering through the work day with the flu, encourage them to go home until the illness has passed. You'll be doing them a favor--they'll recover faster if they get more rest--and also every single other person they may come in contact with by getting them out of the workplace.

Try to Minimize Stress

Stress (https://www.amazon.com/Stress-Your-Health-Recognize-Symptoms/dp/1539766071) is part of daily life and certainly a part of almost every job. But going through extreme stress can burden your immune system and leave you more vulnerable to coming down with colds or the flu. The approach of flu season is a good time to learn or revisit techniques you have for coping with stress.

Practicing positive thinking (https://www.amazon.com/Calm-Mind-Healthy-Discover-Improve/dp/1534774823), giving yourself more encouragement, meditation--any of these methods can help you keep stress at bay and not let it overwhelm you. You may not be able to completely avoid being exposed to flu at work, but you can do things to prevent the virus from attacking you.

Minimize Business Travel

Airplanes and other forms of transportation are closed systems where one person infected with the flu can expose many other people to the disease. If you don't have to travel during cold and flu season, then don't. Try shifting some out of town meetings to teleconferences until spring comes and the danger of flu subsides.

Influenza: Stay Informed and Ready

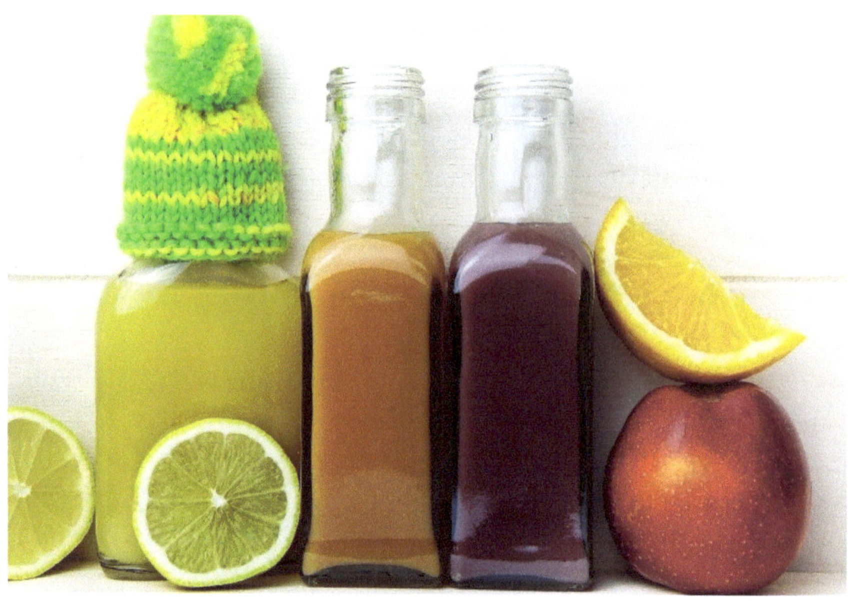

A new strain of flu can pop up any year -- remember the Swine Flu (N1H1) several years ago that swept across the country. Fortunately it had mostly mild, if uncomfortable symptoms. Unfortunately, unlike annual flu, this virus seems to affect younger healthy people with serious consequences including death.

Seasonal flu can cause serious complications for the old and the very young. If you're worried about contracting flu, there are precautions you can take such as washing your hands or using a hand sanitizing gel.

We have so many sources of information available to us these days that it is difficult to sort out what information is credible and which we should disregard.

These three web sites are great tools for flu prevention, coping with the flu after you come down with it, and keeping informed about the scope of this year's influenza outbreak:

- Web Md   www. webmd. com

- Centers for Disease Control www. cdc. gov

- World Health Organization   www. who. int/en/

These websites are constantly updated with new information that you can rely on.

Your state and local health departments also have important information on their websites about areas where the flu outbreak is particularly concentrated, and about schools or other public facilities may be temporarily closed.

For example, a school closure occurred at a prep school in New York after eight students were found to have swine flu. Public health authorities may also provide advice on when to avoid crowds, where flu can be spread easily, when to consider postponing travel, or other social distancing strategies.

The medical community advises that most people should be immunized against the flu every year. However, they also admit that the immunization isn't always effective and that it is possible to get the flu from the immunization if a weakened live flu virus is used instead of a dead virus.

Keep informed by reading the newspaper and watching TV but keep in mind that these days the news media has a tendency to exaggerate bad news and ignore good news.

Planning ahead can help you cope with this situation as well. Make sure you have stocked up on food, medicine, alcohol-based hand rubs, and other supplies you may need should you or your family come down with the flu. Have tea bags, crackers, chicken soup mix, ginger ale, jello, and juices ready to go.

Make sure you have tissues, decongestant spray, and throat lozenges on hand. If you are infected, you need to stay home and take care of yourself, not have to run out to the store where you could infect other people. Being prepared may mean you don't contract influenza flu at all.

Other Relevant Books by This Author

If you would like to read more relevant books about this topic, here is a list of the CreateSpace links, titles and descriptions from this author:

https://www.amazon.com/Stress-Hormone-Cortisol-Chronic-Conditons/dp/153978598X

The Stress Hormone Cortisol: In Chronic Excess, It Can Be the Root Cause of Several Medical Conditions

A person who is under excessive stress is often described as someone who is always working "under the gun". This expression should be a fair indicator that too much exposure to stress is a big threat to a person's health and well-being.

Repeated studies expose the correlation between stress and ill-health, and why chronic stress is such an important health problem. Cortisol is a type of glucocorticoid hormone. Along with adrenaline, it is one of the main hormones responsible for stress responses.

The actions of cortisol in the human body are quite complex. As a primary stress hormone it not only acts directly on the body, but also acts indirectly by activating other hormones, each with a critical role to perform. In a healthy person with a healthy cycle consisting of a stress incident followed by an adequate rest and recovery phase, cortisol has a major function of instigating homeostasis, or returning the body to normal after being exposed to stress.

This is enacted largely through the triggering of secondary hormones. The recovery phase following an acute stress incident is critical for the prevention of developing chronic stress. Chronic stress develops when persistent stress causes stress hormones, including cortisol, to remain constantly elevated in the body. In this all too common situation, cortisol remains awash in the body at high levels for long periods of time.

Unfortunately in today's world, this is happening a lot. In my book, I look not only look at ways to reduce stress, but also some things you can do to better cope with stress.

https://www.amazon.com/Essential-Oils-Health-Healing-Conditions/dp/1542359007

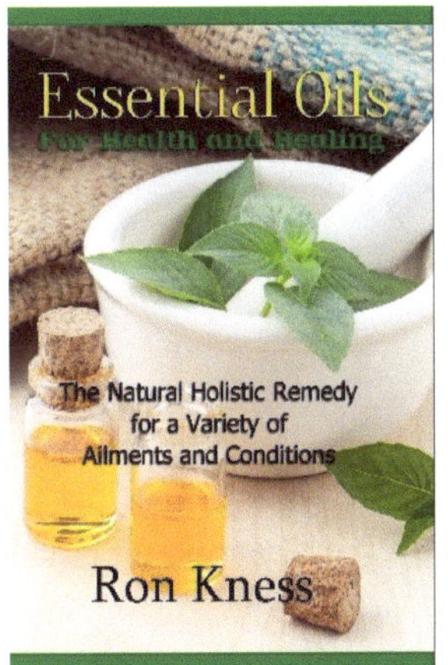

Essential Oils for Health and Healing: The Natural Holistic Remedy for a Variety of Ailments and Conditions

The use of essential oils for therapeutic purposes dates back to 6,000 years ago. The ancient Romans, Indians, Chinese, Greeks, and Egyptians all used them for hygienic, therapeutic, ritualistic, and spiritual purposes.

More than 2,500 years ago, Hippocrates noted that aromatic baths had a significant impact on the overall well-being of an individual. During the early 19th century, essential oils started being present in western medicine practices, while later on in the century, both German and French medical professors started using them to fight infected wounds.

Some of the most popular uses of essential oils are inhalation, massaging essential oils into the skin, and mixing them with face creams and body lotions. By applying essential oils properly, you'll experience a great alternative treatment for stress, fatigue, insomnia and many other health problems. When essential oils are used in a diffuser as aromatherapy, they are well known for improving mood and providing wonderful healing scents that promote general wellness and wellbeing.

Essential oils can not only help you with the health issues noted above, but could end up being your natural holistic remedy for: - Headaches and migraines - Joint aches and pains - Chronic pain - Menstrual irregularities - Cuts, scrapes and burns - Signs of aging and wrinkles - Anxiety and depression If you have never used essential oils before, get a starter kit and start using them. I think you'll be pleasantly surprised at just how beneficial they can be as a natural holistic cure.

https://www.amazon.com/Juicing-Health-Complete-Guide-Nutrition/dp/1533003661

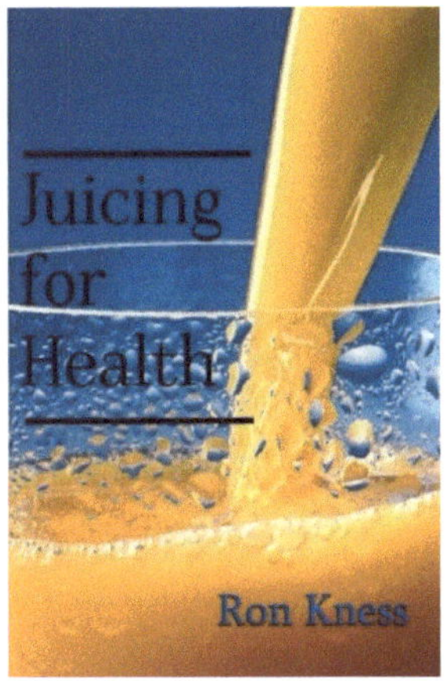

Juicing for Health: The Complete Guide to Juicing for Good Nutrition

It's well documented that many of us need to increase our daily intake of fruit and vegetables. We are the champions of the world when it comes to getting enough of the macronutrients carbs, protein, and fat, but we're sorely lacking when it comes to getting more micronutrients.

While the Centers For Disease Control recommend adults consume about 1 ½ to 2 cups of fruit and 2 to 3 cups of vegetables daily, an analysis of American diets between 2007 and 2010 found that 50% of the population ate less than 1 cup of fruit and less than 1 ½ cups of vegetables. An astounding 76% of people did not eat nearly enough fruit, and 87% did not eat enough vegetables.

Many people simply don't like eating vegetables. Broccoli is tough, cabbage is chewy, and carrots can break your teeth if they haven't been boiled long enough and let's not get started on that stringy asparagus!

However, fruit and vegetables are where essential micronutrients are to be found and juicing is a great way to easily pack more of them into a well-balanced and healthy diet. Thousands have joined the juicing revolution and for good reason, it is healthy, convenient and allows you to get key vitamins and minerals from plant foods that may be missing from your diet.

About the Author

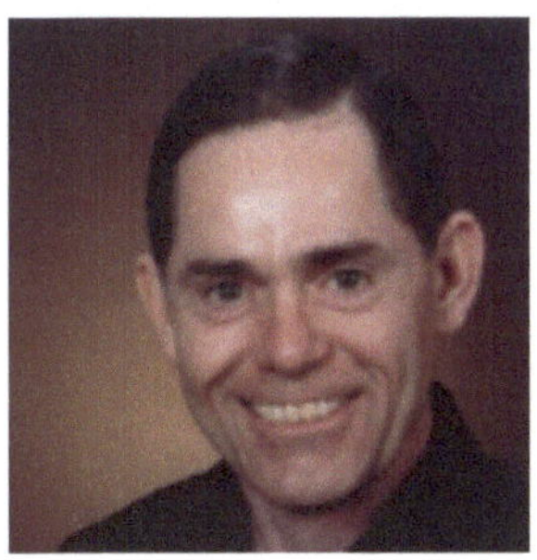

I have published over 125 books on Amazon for Kindle, CreateSpace and other publishing platforms.

While most of my books are on health and fitness in general, as I age (now 65) at the time of this writing) my topics of interest are geared toward aging baby boomers and older.

Besides my own writing, I also ghostwrite ebooks, books, reports, articles, blogs and do Kindle conversions for clients on a variety of topics.

Today my wife and I are retired from our careers and live in Gold Canyon, AZ. I now write as a retirement business where you'll find me happily sitting in my office typing away on my laptop as I work on my next book or ghostwriting project . . . that is if we are not traveling on a cruise ship - our new-found mode of travel.

9 781983 656002